Protein Bars At Home

DIY Protein Bar Recipes For A Healthier Life

Ariana Hunter

© 2015

Table of Contents

Introduction

Greetings! Thank for choosing to read my book. You are about to enter into the world of healthy, mouthwatering, and easy-to-make DIY protein bars! You will learn about protein bars, the many types of protein powders available to you, and you will definitely enjoy some tasty recipes.

The information is this book is easy to follow and understand. You can mix and match ingredients and experiment with the recipes at your own discretion. However, it's likely that you won't find the need to tinker with the recipes at all. Not only are these protein bars cost efficient, but many of the protein bars in this book taste 10 times better than what you'll find in any store. Some of the recipes in this book include, baked protein bars, no-bake protein bars, low-carb/low-calories protein bars, and vegan protein bars.

Protein bars, while they are helpful, should only be considered as a supplementary component of your diet. Relying on protein bars as the main source of your food intake can deny you the benefits of the much-needed minerals, vitamins, fiber, healthy fats, and phytochemicals that are abundant in other foods. As long you have a healthy and balanced diet, consuming protein bars shouldn't need to be a daily occurrence. Your main focus should be nutrition and proper exercise. If you are looking for a product to help you lose weight, gain muscle or add more protein to your diet without the added calories, then protein bars are the best choice. But only use them as a supplement and not a meal.

Some protein powders can contain as much protein as your regular chicken breast. Most manufacturers of protein powders use soy or whey protein as the main ingredient. Let's take a dive into the wonderful world of protein bars so that you can learn 31 amazing recipes and start to save money but making your own healthy protein bars.

Chapter 1 – What Are Protein Bars?

Protein is necessary to build, maintain and repair muscle. To increase protein in your diet, you could turn to meats, which are complete protein sources because they provide all the needed amino acids. The downside to meats, especially red meat, is that they can also provide significant amounts of saturated fat and cholesterol. Another way to increase protein intake is by combining servings of incomplete proteins such as legumes and grains, but this can increase carbohydrate and calorie intake. Some powders and drinks can offer a protein alternative without significantly increasing consumption of fats, carbohydrates, cholesterol or calories!

Advantages
Energy bars are delicious, convenient, and healthy. Most contain moderate amounts of fat, and sodium. Many are a good source of high quality protein without the cholesterol and saturated fat of high fat animal protein sources. They have a low amount of sodium, but most are packed with vitamins and minerals. In short, for a small meal or snack they are a better choice than a fast food meal and other highly processed packaged convenience foods.

Disadvantages
Even though protein bars are fortified with the same mineral and vitamins and vegetables and fruits, they do not contain the phytochemicals, organic fiber, bioflavonoids, and balance of vitamins and minerals that are found in these foods. A lot of protein bars do not even come close to containing the amount of fiber that you would normally find in whole grains, beans, or any other carbohydrates.

Chapter 2 – The Benefits of Making Your Own Protein Bars

Even though store-bought protein bars claim to carry many benefits, they are loaded with sugar and unhealthy artificial sweeteners. The carbs and calories in these protein bars are very low, but in reality, consuming these bars in large quantities can cause a number of side effects. These side effects include, but are not limited to flatulence, bloating, and maybe even diarrhea.

Most health enthusiasts and athletes depend on protein to assist the body in building muscle. Some might turn to these unhealthy protein bars to assist them, but the body does not perform at its best using unhealthy, artificial sugars and carbohydrates. In addition to other nutrients, the human body needs protein to build muscle. In the fitness and medical fields it is generally accepted that protein after exercise helps build and repair muscle.

Homemade protein bars are a better choice because you will be getting the sweetness and sugar from natural sources like fruit, which has been proven to be a better choice for athletic performance and endurance. The body needs healthy sugars to perform at a healthy and stable rate.

These protein bars really do contain plenty of protein from high-quality, low-sugar protein powders that carry some of the best sources of protein that the body needs. An added bonus is that the ingredients like, yogurt, oats, flaxseed, peanut butter, almond butter, almonds, walnuts, peanuts, chia seeds, apricots and other ingredients are very reliable sources of healthy sugars, carbs, and proteins.

The beauty is that you don't always need to bake these protein bars, and you can add as much protein as you like. You will find also that you will feel a lot better by eating them.

Chapter 3 – The Best Protein Powders

Protein is a macronutrient that can be found in many foods such as meats, dairy products, nuts, and beans. Protein is made up of amino acids, which are the building blocks of lean body tissue.

The main ingredient in protein bars is protein powder. There is a number of various protein powders on the market that you can choose from to add to your protein bars. Let's take a look at some of the basic information about these bars, so you can make the decision on which one is best for you.

It may be shocking to find that some of the protein powders that you can buy at your local health food store or vitamin shop may not be the right one for the goal you are trying to reach. All protein powders are not created equal. It is important to have a clear understanding of your goals and the protein powder that will help you reach those goals successfully. Sometimes carelessly picking out protein powders can cause you to have some unforeseen health issues. So, it's important to always read the labels and it's always best to do some research on different protein powders, and figure out how they can benefit you and your goal. This will make it easier for you to stick with what you know. Instead of going through the anxiety of sticking to what you don't.

Protein Isolate, Concentrate and Hydrolysate
Protein can be found in varying food products, meats, and produce. The protein found in your favorite protein powders has likely gone through some of the following processes:

Isolated Protein – This will be the more expensive protein type. It is created through a process called protein purification. This process isolates protein from a specific organism, and is composed of a higher percentage of pure protein. The best qualities of isolate protein are usually free of fat, cholesterol, carbs, and lactose.

Concentrated Protein – This is the least expensive form of protein and is usually derived from cheese. This protein usually has lower levels of carbs, fat, and cholesterol, with only a weight of 30% to 90% protein.

Hydrolyzed Protein – This type of protein is processed by protein hydrolysis. This process involves breaking the protein down into its key amino acids.

What Type to Use?
There are five main types of protein powders on the market today. Most people choose to buy casein, soy, whey, or rice protein. Here is a list of different protein powders to choose from, and a little information about them.

Whey

This fast-digesting protein is made up of a mixture of globular proteins that are isolated from whey or the byproduct of cheese. This protein is ideal to consume right before a workout. New to the market, some consider whey protein as one of the highest quality proteins available on the market.

Paleo

This protein is ideal for Paleo dieters, bodybuilders, cross-trainers, and athletes. All of the ingredients in Paleo protein is natural and packed with muscle building proteins. Paleo powder is sugar free, lactose free, gluten free, and fat free.

Casein

Casein is a slower digesting protein, and is the ideal choice when you are in between meals, or would like to have something as a meal replacement. This protein powder is special because it has the ability to form a gel or clot in the stomach, allowing the nutrients and amino acids to be released slowly while it is being digested.

Soy

Made from soybean meal, soy protein is the most popular choice for vegetarians and vegans. The protein is isolated from beans that have been hulled and the fat has been extracted from them. The end result is usually a powder that is made up of 70% protein and 20% carbs.

Pea Protein

The great thing about pea protein is that it is high in Lysine. Lysine is responsible for converting fatty acids into energy that assist the body in lowering cholesterol and calcium absorption. It also plays a key role in producing collagen which is the main component for healthy skin, bones, tendons, and connective tissue. Lysine is not naturally produced by the human body, and cannot be produced unless in the body and must therefore be consumed through the diet.

Chapter 4 – Weight Loss Protein Bars

These weight loss protein bars are sure to help you keep your waistline in check. You'll be eligible for seconds with these.

Vanilla-Buttermilk Protein Bar

Yield: Twelve Bars
Active Time: 15 minutes
Cooking Time: 45 minutes
Total Time: 1 hour

Ingredients
Crust:
- ⅔ cup almond flour
- 2 tbsp coconut flour
- ¼ cup monk fruit sweetener
- ⅛ tsp Himalayan Pink salt
- Unrefined Himalayan Pink salt

Filling:
- 8 scoops Soy Protein Powder (Vanilla Flavor)
- ½ cup monk sweetener
- 2 large eggs, lightly beaten
- ¾ cup buttermilk
- 2 tbsp butter, melted
- 3 tbsp organic raw honey
- 2 tbsp coconut flour
- 2 tsp lime peel
- 2 tsp orange peel, freshly grated
- ½ tsp vanilla extract

Cooking Directions
1. Set oven to 350 degrees, and lightly grease an 8"x8" baking pan with coconut oil.
2. In a large bowl, beat together butter and sweetener until the mixture becomes creamy using an electric mixer. Add flour and salt and mix on low speed until all ingredients are thoroughly blended.
3. Pour the batter into the prepared baking dish, and spread evenly and press to encourage a crust. Place in the oven to bake for a minimum of 15 to 20 minutes.
4. In the meantime, beat together eggs and sugar in a large bowl using an electric mixer. Slowly mix in butter, honey, corn syrup, flour, protein powder, vanilla, lime

peel, and orange peel. Mix until the mixture reaches a smooth consistency. Pour filling over the crust.

5. Place in the oven to bake for a minimum of 20 to 25 minutes or until the edges of the crust begin to brown and the filling is set. Remove from the oven and allow the batter to cool, and cut into 12 bars when ready to serve.

Low-Calorie Fudge Bar

Yield: Eight Bars
Active Time: 5 minutes
Cooking Time: 0 minutes
Total Time: 1 hour, 5 minutes

Ingredients
- 8 tbsp Casein Protein Powder (Chocolate)
- 1 ½ cup black beans, cooked, and drained
- 3 tbsp cacao powder
- ⅔ cup chocolate chips
- ⅓ cup organic raw honey
- 2 tbsp monk fruit sweetener
- 1 tbsp baking powder
- 3 ½ tbsp unrefined virgin coconut oil
- ¼ tsp Himalayan Pink salt

Ingredients
1. Set oven to 350 degrees, and lightly grease an 8"x8" baking pan with coconut oil.
2. In a large blender or food processor, mix together all ingredients, excluding the chocolate chips. Mix in chocolate chips and pour into the prepared baking dish. Press and pat down using a rubber spatula to even out the batter in the pan.
3. Place in the oven to bake for a minimum of 17 minutes or until the batter is set. Remove from the oven and allow batter to cool for overnight or for a minimum of 8 hours. Cut into 10 bars when ready to serve. Store remainder in an airtight container.

Low-Carb Nutty Bar

Yield: Eight Bars
Active Time: 5 minutes
Cooking Time: 0 minutes
Total Time: 1 hour, 5 minutes

Ingredients
- 4 scoops Hydrolyzed Protein Powder (Peanut Butter Flavor)
- 1 ½ cup rolled-oats
- 1 cup almond butter
- ¼ cup unsweetened applesauce
- ¾ cup dried cranberries
- ¾ cup silvered almonds, chopped
- ½ cup pistachios, chopped
- ⅓ cup pumpkin seeds
- ⅓ cup ground flaxseeds
- ⅓ cup walnuts, chopped
- ¼ cup sunflower seeds
- ⅓ cup organic raw honey

Directions
1. Line an 8"x8" baking dish with parchment paper and set to the side.
2. In a large bowl, combine protein powder, oats, almonds, cranberries, pistachios, flaxseed, walnuts, pumpkin seeds, and sunflower seeds. Stir in applesauce, almond butter, and honey, and mix well to combine.
3. Pour into a prepared baking dish and press down using a rubber spatula. Place in freezer and chill for a minimum of 1 hour or until the batter has set.
4. Cut into 8 bars when ready to serve, and store the leftovers in an airtight container.

Low-Carb High-Protein Cinnamon and Apple Bars

Yield: Sixteen Bars
Active Time: 25 minutes
Cooking Time: 0 minutes
Total Time: 4 hours, 5 minutes

Ingredients
- 4 scoops Hydrolyzed Protein Powder (Vanilla Flavor)
- 1 large green apple, peeled, cored, and grated
- ½ cup almond meal
- 3 large eggs, lightly beaten
- ½ cup cottage cheese
- ¼ cup monk fruit sweetener
- 2 tsp baking powder
- ¼ tsp nutmeg
- ¼ tsp allspice
- 2 tsp ground cinnamon
- 1 tsp almond extract
- Unrefined virgin coconut oil

Cooking Directions
1. Set oven to 350 degrees, and lightly grease an 8"x8" baking sheet. Set to the side.
2. In a large bowl, combine protein powder, almond meal, baking powder, cinnamon, nutmeg, allspice, and salt. Beat together using a fork or a whisk. Form a well in the center.
3. In a separate bowl, combine eggs, sweetener, cheese, and almond extract. Beat together using a whisk, and pour into the dry ingredients. Mix well to combine, and gently fold in apples.
4. Pour into the prepared baking dish and bake for a minimum of 25 minutes. Remove from the baking pan from oven and allow the batter to cool. Cut into 8 bars when ready to serve. Store any remainder in an airtight container.

Almond Cheesecake Protein Bars

Yield: Twenty Servings
Active Time: 15 minutes
Cooking Time: 1 hour
Total Time: 1 hour, 15 minutes

Ingredients
- 6 scoops Paleo Protein Powder (Vanilla-Almond)
- 1 cup almond butter, melted
- 12 ounces cream cheese
- ¼ cup organic coconut cream concentrate
- 2 large eggs, lightly beaten
- ¼ cup silvered almonds, sliced
- ¼ cup silvered almonds, finely ground (divided)
- 1 ¼ cup vanilla wafer crumbs
- ¼ cup monk fruit sweetener
- ⅓ cup light butter, melted
- 1 tsp coconut extract
- 2 ½ tsp almond extract
- ½ cup organic raw honey
- Unrefined virgin coconut oil

Cooking Directions
1. Set oven to 350 degrees, and lightly grease an 8"x8" baking dish with coconut oil.
2. In a large bowl, combine vanilla wafers, butter, ground almonds, and sweetener. Press into the prepared pan and press down using rubber spatula to encourage crust. Bake in the oven for a minimum of 10 to 15 minutes. Pour melted almond butter over the pie crust, and spread around to the edges. Set to the side.
3. In a large bowl, combine protein powder, cream cheese, honey, eggs, almond extract, coconut extract, and coconut cream. Beat together using an electric mixer at medium spread, and pour over the prepared crust. Place in the oven and bake for a minimum of 40 to 45 minutes, or until the cheesecake becomes firm.
4. Remove the cheesecake from the oven, top with sliced almonds, and allow the cheesecakes to cool. Cut into 20 bars when ready to serve, and store remaining in an airtight container.

Chewy Peanut Butter Bars

Yield: Six Bars
Active Time: 5 minutes
Cooking Time: 0 minutes
Total Time: 4 hours, 5 minutes

Ingredients
- 10 tbsp Paleo Protein Power (Vanilla-Almond)
- 3 tbsp carob powder
- 2 tbsp sesame seeds
- ½ cup ground flaxseed
- 2 tbsp coconut flour
- ⅓ cup organic coconut peanut butter
- ½ cup coconut water
- ⅛ tsp organic raw honey
- 1 tsp almond extract
- 2 tbsp unrefined virgin coconut oil

Cooking Directions
1. Lightly grease a 9"x9" baking dish.
2. Mix together protein powder, carob powder, flaxseed, flour, and sesame seeds. Form a well in the center.
3. In a small saucepan, mix together peanut butter and coconut oil. Cook for a minimum of 5 minutes. Pour into the dry ingredients. Stir until the ingredients are dry and crumbly. Add water and almond extract. Mix well to blend. Pour into prepared baking dish.
4. Place in the fridge to set for a minimum of 4 hours, and cut into 6 bars when ready to serve.

Low-Calorie Cranberry Banana Oatmeal Bars

Yield: Eight Bars
Active Time: 10 minutes
Cooking Time: 25 minutes
Total Time: 50 minutes

Ingredients
- ⅔ cup Casein Protein Powder (Vanilla Powder)
- 2 tbsp chia seeds
- 2 cups bananas, mashed
- 2 cups rolled-oats
- ¼ cup hibiscus tea, brewed
- ½ cup silvered almonds, chopped
- ½ cup almond butter, softened
- ½ cup craisins
- ½ cup coconut flakes, shredded
- 1 ½ tsp ground cinnamon
- 1 tsp vanilla extract
- Unrefined virgin olive oil

Cooking Directions
1. Set oven to 350 degrees, and lightly grease an 8"x8" baking pan. Set to the side.
2. Combine oats, banana, almond butter, protein powder, craisins, coconut, chia seeds, tea, almonds, cinnamon, and vanilla. Pour and spread into the prepared pan.
3. Place in the oven to bake for a minimum of 25 to 30 minutes. Allow the batter to cool for a minimum of 15 minutes. Cut into 8 bars before servings.

Low-Calorie Peanut Butter and Apricot Jelly Bars

Yield: Eight Bars
Active Time: 5 minutes
Cooking Time: 20 minutes
Total Time: 25 minutes

Ingredients
- ½ cup Hydrolyzed Protein Powder (Vanilla Flavor)
- ¼ cup PB2
- 2 tbsp unsweetened applesauce
- ¼ cup almond milk
- ¼ cup egg whites
- ¼ cup monk fruit sweetener
- ½ cup apricot preserves
- ½ tsp baking powder
- ¼ tsp Himalayan Pink salt
- Unrefined virgin coconut oil

Cooking Directions
1. Set oven to 350 degrees, and lightly grease a loaf pan with coconut oil. Set to the side.
2. In a large bowl, combine protein powder, PB2, applesauce, almond milk, egg whites, sweetener, baking powder, and salt. Mix well until all ingredients are well combined. Pour into the prepared loaf pan, pour apricot preserves into the batter and mix in using a rubber spatula.
3. Place in the oven to bake for a minimum of 15 to 20 minutes or until the batter sets and is lightly browned. Remove from oven and allow cool. Cut into 8 bars before serving. Store remainder in an airtight container.

Low-Calories Protein Blondies

Yield: Six Bars
Active Time: 10 minutes
Cooking Time: 15 minutes
Total Time: 1 hour, 5 minutes

Ingredients
- 4 scoops Paleo Protein Powder (Vanilla-Almond)
- 2 tbsp sunflower seeds
- 4 tbsp ground flaxseeds
- 2 large eggs, lightly beaten
- 4 tsp monk fruit sweetener
- ¼ cup unrefined virgin olive oil

Cooking Directions
1. Set oven to 350 degrees, lightly grease a 5"x3" baking dish with coconut oil.
2. Using clean hands, combine all ingredients in a large bowl, and dump into prepared baking dish. Bake for a minimum of 15 minutes or until the batter is lightly browned.

Chapter 5 – Baked Protein Bars

These baked goods are full of mean protein, and you will be sure to enjoy these as a tasty pre-workout snack or a healthy dessert.

Gooey Lemon Protein Bars

Yield: Thirty-Six Bars
Active Time: 25 minutes
Cooking Time: 35 minutes
Total Time: 3 hours, 30 minutes

Ingredients
- 10 scoops Whey Protein Powder (Vanilla Flavor)
- 2 cup almond flour
- ¼ cup coconut flour
- 2 cups monk fruit sweetener
- 1 cup butter, softened
- ½ cup lemon juice, freshly squeezed
- 4 large eggs, lightly beaten
- ½ tsp baking powder
- 3 tsp lime zest, freshly grated
- Himalayan Pink salt, to taste
- Unrefined virgin coconut oil

Cooking Directions
1. Set oven to 350 degrees, and lightly grease a 12"x15" baking dish with coconut oil.
2. In a large bowl, mix together 4 scoops of protein powder and almond flour. Cut in butter until the mixture become crumbly. Press into the bottom of the bottom of the prepared baking dish. Place in the oven and allow the batter to bake for a minimum of 10 minutes or until the crust is very lightly browned.
3. In the meantime, beat together eggs ⅓ cup lemon juice, coconut flour, sweetener, lemon zest, and baking powder. Pour over the crust, and return to the oven to bake for a minimum of 25 minutes. Remove from oven and cool for a minimum of 30 minutes.
4. In a large bowl, mix together 2 tablespoons of lemon juice and remaining protein powder. Spread evenly over the cooled lemon bars. Allow the glaze to set.

Cheat-Day Super Sweet Hawaiian Protein Bars

Yield: Thirty-Six Servings
Active Time: 10 minutes
Cooking Time: 50 minutes
Total Time: 1 hour

Ingredients
- 8 scoops Raw Whey Protein Powder.
- 1 (17.5 ounce) package organic sugar cookie mix
- 1 cup dried pineapple, coarsely chopped
- 2 cups peanut butter chips
- 1 cup sweetened coconut flakes, shredded
- ½ cup silvered almonds, finely chopped
- 1 cup macadamia nuts, chopped
- 2 cups vanilla almond milk
- 1 egg, lightly beaten
- ½ cup butter or margarine, softened
- Unrefined virgin coconut oil

Directions
1. Set oven to 350 degrees, and lightly grease a 9"x13" baking dish with coconut oil.
2. Combine cookie mix, protein powder, butter, milk, and egg in a large bowl. Mix well until a smooth and soft cookie dough forms. Press cookie dough into the bottom of the prepared baking dish.
3. Bake for 15 minutes and remove from oven. Pour in vanilla baking chips, pineapple, coconut, almonds, and macadamia onto the baked cookie crust. Tops with milk. Bake until mixture is light golden brown or for 30 to 35 minutes. Remove from oven and allow casserole to cool. Cut into 9x4 rows when ready to serve. Store remainder of bars in an airtight container.

Ginger Crunch Protein Bars

Yield: Eight Bars
Active Time: 5 minutes
Cooking Time: 20 minutes
Total Time: 25 minutes

Ingredients
- 2 scoops Isolate Soy Protein Powder (Vanilla Flavor)
- 1 ½ cups apple cinnamon protein cereal, crushed
- 1 cup rolled oats
- ½ cup crystallized ginger, chopped (divided)
- ¼ cup sweetened coconut, shredded
- ¼ cup sunflower seeds
- ¼ cup full-fat coconut milk
- ¼ cup organic raw honey
- 2 tbsp butter, melted

Cooking Directions
1. Set oven to 325 degrees, and line a 9"x9" baking dish with parchment paper. Set to the side.
2. In a medium saucepan, stir together butter, honey, milk, and protein powder. Beat together until smooth. Remove from heat and keep warm.
3. In a large bowl, stir together cereal, oats, almonds, sunflower seeds, and ⅜ cup crystallized ginger. Slowly stir butter mixture. Mix well to combine all ingredients.
4. Pour batter onto prepared baking dish. Press and spread batter out evenly using a rubber spatula. Top with remaining ginger and coconut.
5. Place in the oven to bake for a minimum of 20 minutes or until the batter has set. Remove from oven and cool. Cut into 8 bars when ready to serve. Store remaining bars in an airtight container.

Vanilla Farina Bars

Yield: Twelve Bars
Active Time: 10 minutes
Cooking Time: 45 minutes
Total Time: 1 hour, 5 minutes

Ingredients
- 3 scoops Isolate Soy Protein Powder (Vanilla)
- ½ cup sweet coconut flakes
- 2 cup dry cream of wheat
- ¼ cup unsweetened applesauce
- 1 cup organic Greek yogurt
- ½ cup silvered almonds, sliced
- ¼ cup butter, softened
- ½ cup 100% pure cane sugar
- ⅓ cup organic raw honey
- 2 tbsp lemon zest
- 2 tsp baking powder
- 1tsp cardamom
- 1 tsp almond extract
- Unrefined virgin coconut oil

Cooking Directions
1. Set oven to 350 degrees, and lightly grease a 9"x13" baking dish with coconut oil.
2. In a large bowl, cream butter, applesauce, sugar, and honey using an electric mixer. Beat in lemon juice.
3. In a separate bowl, combine coconut flakes, almonds, protein powder, cream of wheat, cardamom, and baking powder. Form a well in the center and pour sugar mixture into the center. Beat in eggs and yogurt using an electric mixer at medium speed. Mix until a smooth consistency is reached. Be careful not to overmix.
4. Pour mixture into the pan and smooth using a rubber spatula.
5. Place in the oven to bake for a minimum of 45 to 55 minutes or until the edges of the batter have browned.
6. Remove from the oven and cool. Cut into twelve bars when ready to serve. Store the remainder of the bars in an airtight container

Vanilla Lime Protein Bars

Yield: Thirty-Two Bars
Active Time: 15 minutes
Cooking Time: 40 minutes
Total Time: 55 minutes

Ingredients
- ¼ cup Whey Isolate Protein (Vanilla Flavor)
- 2 tsp Matcha Green Tea Powder
- ½ cup lime juice, freshly squeezed
- 1 ¾ cup 100% pure cane sugar
- 2 cups almond flour
- 4 tbsp coconut flour
- 4 eggs, lightly beaten
- 1 cup butter, softened
- ½ cup organic raw honey
- Unrefined virgin coconut oil

Cooking Directions
1. Set oven to 350 degrees, and lightly a 9"x13" baking dish with coconut oil, and set to the side.
2. In a large bowl, stir together mix together 2 cups flour, Matcha Green Tea Powder, and ½ cup sugar. Mix well together to combine. Cut in butter and mix well to blend. Press the batter down into the bottom of the prepared baking dish. Place in the oven to bake for a minimum of 15 to 20 minutes or until the crust becomes golden. Remove from heat and set to the side.
3. In a separate bowl, beat together remaining sugar and ¼ cup flours, eggs, and lemon juice. Pour on top of the baked crust.
4. Place in the oven to bake for a minimum of 20 minutes. Remove from oven and allow the lime bars to cool and firm. Serve immediately and store remainder in an airtight container.

Chewy High-Protein Granola Bars

Yield: Twelve Bars
Active Time: 10 minutes
Cooking Time: 20 minutes
Total Time: 30 minutes

Ingredients
- ½ cup Paleo Protein powder (Vanilla Flavor)
- 2 cups organic rolled-oats
- 2 tbsp ground flaxseed
- ⅓ cup cacao nibs
- 2 tbsp chocolate chips
- ¼ cup organic coconut peanut butter
- ½ cup almond milk (vanilla flavor)
- ¼ cup organic raw honey
- 1 tsp coconut extract
- ¼ tsp Himalayan Pink salt
- Unrefined virgin coconut oil

Cooking Directions
1. Set oven to 350 degrees, and lightly grease a, 8"x8" baking sheet with coconut oil.
2. Combine protein powder, oats, flax, cinnamon, and salt. Mix well to combine, form a well in the center of the ingredients, and set to the side.
3. In a separate bowl, stir together almond butter, honey, almond milk, and coconut extract. Blend well and pour into the well of the dry ingredients. Stir until all of the ingredients are incorporated, and there is a smooth consistency. Gently fold in cacao nibs and chocolate chips, and pour onto the prepared baking dish. Spread batter out evenly using a rubber spatula. Press down the batter.
4. Place in the oven to bake for a minimum of 20 minutes or until the batter has set. Remove from the oven and allow the granola to cool for a minimum to 20 minutes. Cut into 12 bars before serving. Store remainder in an airtight container.

Hazelnut Cacao Bars

Yield: Twelve Bars
Active Time: 5 minutes
Cooking Time: 21 minutes
Total Time: 1 hour, 26 minutes

Ingredients
- 3 tbsp Hemp Protein Powder
- 2 cups cacao nibs
- ¼ cup hazelnuts, chopped
- ½ cup walnuts, chopped
- ⅓ cup dried cherries, coarsely chopped
- 2 tbsp crystallized ginger, finely chopped
- Unrefined virgin olive oil

Cooking Directions
1. Set oven to 350 degrees. Line a baking sheet with foil, and set to the side.
2. Place hazelnuts on a baking sheet and roast for 20 minutes, stirring once after first 10 minutes. Remove from oven and allow hazelnuts to cool. Dump nuts out onto a towel. Roll up towel to gently rub against hazelnuts to remove skin, and coarsely chop nuts.
3. In a medium bowl, combine nuts, ginger, hemp protein, and cherries. Toss gently to combine.
4. Place nibs in a microwave-safe measuring cup, and microwave at HIGH for 60 seconds or until chocolate melts, stirring every 15 seconds.
5. Add melted chocolate to nut mixture, stirring until combined nut mixture is well coated. Spread mixture evenly on prepared baking sheet and freeze 1 hour. Break into 1 ounce pieces once chocolate is set and serve immediately.

Nut Butter Protein Bars

Yield: Sixteen Bars
Active Time: 10 minutes
Cooking Time: 20 minutes
Total Time: 30 minutes

Ingredients
- 2 scoops Soy Protein Chocolate (Chocolate Flavor)
- ½ cup chocolate chips
- 1 cup rolled-oats
- 1 cup sweet shredded coconut
- ¼ cup almond butter
- ¼ cup coconut peanut butter
- ¾ cup peanuts, chopped
- ½ cup almond milk (Chocolate Flavor)
- ¼ cup organic raw honey
- 2 tsp almond extract
- ¼ tsp Himalayan Pink, salt
- Unrefined virgin coconut oil

Cooking Directions
1. Set oven to 350 degrees, and lightly grease a, 8"x8" baking sheet with coconut oil.
2. In a large saucepan, over medium-high heat mix together honey, almond butter, peanut butter, and coconut oil. Mix well until all ingredients are combined. Set to the side and keep warm. Remove from heat and mix in chocolate chips.
3. Combine protein powder, oats, shredded coconut, and salt. Mix well to combine, form a well in the center of the ingredients, and set to the side.
4. In a separate bowl, stir together almond butter, honey, almond milk, and almond extract. Blend well and pour into the well of the dry ingredients. Stir until all of the ingredients are incorporated, and there is a smooth consistency. Gently fold in cacao nibs and chocolate chips, and pour onto the prepared baking dish. Spread batter into out evenly using a rubber spatula. Press down the batter.
5. Place in the oven to bake for a minimum of 20 minutes or until the batter has set. Remove from the oven and allow the granola to cool for a minimum to 20 minutes. Drizzle caramel over the top of the caramel bars. Cut into 12 bars before serving.

High-Protein Peanut Butter Chocolate Cheesecake Bars

Yield: Twenty Bars
Active Time: 15 minutes
Cooking Time: 1 hour
Total Time: 4 hour, 15 minutes

Ingredients
- ½ cup Casein Protein (Vanilla Flavored)
- ¾ cup coconut peanut butter
- 1 cup peanut butter chips
- 1 cup chocolate chips
- 1 ¼ cups whole-wheat graham cracker crumbs
- 1 ½ cups raw almonds, finely chopped
- ¼ cup caramel
- 32 ounces cream cheese, softened
- 4 large eggs
- ¼ cup egg white
- ⅓ cup butter
- 1 cup organic raw honey (divided)
- 2 tsp almond extract

Cooking Directions
1. Set oven to 350 degrees, and lightly grease a 9"x9" baking dish with olive oil and set to the side.
2. Add almonds, graham cracker crumbs, and butter to a food processor and blend until the dough sticks together. Dump graham dough into the prepared baking dish, and press mixture down firmly to encourage crust. Brush with egg white. Bake mixture in the oven for 5 minutes. Remove from oven and aside to cool.
3. Using an electric mixer, beat cream cheese, peanut butter, almond butter, and honey together in a large bowl. Gradually add eggs, coconut cream, and coconut extract. Continue to beat until cream mixture is smooth. Gently fold in peanut butter chips, chocolate chips, and protein powder dump mixture onto crust. Evenly distribute and spread with a rubber spatula.
4. Bake for a minimum of 50 to 55 minutes, or until firm mixture is set and firm. Remove from oven and cool on a wire rack for 30 minutes. Cover with plastic wrap and place in fridge to chill for 2 hours.
5. When cheesecake is set, combine caramel and walnuts a small saucepan, and melt caramel over medium heat. Stirring constantly, spread melted caramel and nuts over cheesecake, cut into 12 bars, and serve immediately.

Chapter 6 – No Bake Protein Bars

No need to bake these protein bars, as they are made without an oven, and are composed of healthy ingredients. However, that's more time for you to spend in the gym.

German Chocolate Cacao Bars

Yield: Twelve Bars
Active Time: 20 minutes
Chilling Time: 2 hours
Total Time: 2 hours, 20 minutes

Ingredients
- ½ cup Soy Protein Powder (Chocolate Flavor)
- ½ cup rolled oats, processed to a fine flour
- 1 cup dates, pitted and chopped
- ¾ cup pecans, chopped (**divided**)
- ¾ cup sweetened coconut flakes, shredded (divided)
- 2 tbsp chocolate chips
- ¼ cup cacao powder (divided)
- ¼ cup coconut water
- 1 tsp vanilla extract
- ½ tsp Himalayan Pink salt

Directions
1. Line an 8"x8" baking dish with parchment paper.
2. Combine rolled oats, ½ cup coconut, ½ cup pecans, cacao powder, dates, vanilla, water, and protein powder in a food processor. Process until the ingredients form into dough. Dump into a large bowl, and mix in remaining pecans, ⅛ cup cacao powder, and chocolate chips. Pour ingredients into a prepared baking dish.
3. Place in the fridge to set for a minimum of 2 to 3 hours to set. Cut into 12 bars when ready to serve. Store remaining bars in an airtight container.

No-Bake Coconut Butter Bars

Yield: Eight Bars
Active Time: 15 minutes
Cooking Time: 5 minutes
Chilling Time: 20 minutes
Total Time: 40 minutes

Ingredients
- 1 cup Soy Protein (Chocolate Flavor)
- ⅓ cup silvered almonds, finely chopped
- 2 tbsp chia seeds
- ¾ cup organic coconut peanut butter
- 1 cup organic full-fat coconut milk
- 1 cup coconut flour
- 1 cup rice cereal
- ¼ cup tbsp cacao nibs
- 3 tbsp chocolate chip
- 2 tbsp coconut water
- 4 tbsp organic raw honey
- 1 tsp coconut extract

Cooking Directions
1. Place parchment paper in an 8"x8" baking dish, and set to the side.
2. Combine flour, protein powder, almonds, cereal, and chia seeds and form a well in the center of the ingredients.
3. In a large saucepan, mix together milk, honey, and coconut peanut butter. Allow to cook for a minimum of 5 minutes or until the mixture becomes slightly runny. Remove from heat and add cacao nibs stir until the cacao nibs melt. Pour into the well of the dry ingredients and mix well to combines. Add coconut water and continue to stir.
4. Dump mixture into lined baking dish and press the batter down to pack, using a rubber spatula or clean hands. Place in the freezer to set for a minimum of 20 minutes or longer.
5. When ready to serve but into eight bars. Store excess in an airtight container and place in the fridge or freezer.

High-Protein Coconut Date Bars

Yield: Six Bars
Active Time: 10 minutes
Chilling Time: 30 minutes
Total Time: 40 minutes

Ingredients
- 3 scoops Paleo Protein Powder
- ⅓ cups organic silvered almonds
- ½ cup organic coconut flakes
- 10 dates, pitted
- ¼ cup organic cashews
- 1 tsp organic unrefined virgin coconut oil

Directions
1. Line a large baking sheet with parchment paper, and set to the side.
2. Add almonds and coconut flakes to a blender, and blend until the almond, protein powder, and coconut are pulverized. Dump in the dates and blend until the mixture is combined. Finally, add the cashews and coconut oil and blend until the mixture thickens and becomes sticky.
3. Pour the mixture onto the parchment lined baking sheet, and form the batter into a square. Fold the sides of the parchment paper over the top of the batter.
4. Place the batter into the fridge, and allow the batter to chill for about 30 minutes before serving.

Hemp & Pumpkin Protein Bars

Yield: Sixteen Bars
Active Time: 20 minutes
Chilling Time: 2 hours
Total Time: 2 hours, 20 minutes

Ingredients
- 2 scoops Whey Protein Powders
- ½ cup dates, pitted, and chopped
- ½ cup hemp seed butter
- 2 cups rolled-oats
- ¼ cup raw pumpkin seeds
- 2 tbsp chia seeds
- ½ cup rose water
- ¼ cup organic raw honey
- ½ tsp coconut extract
- ½ tsp cinnamon
- ¼ tsp nutmeg
- Himalayan Pink salt, to taste

Directions
1. Place parchment paper in an 8"x8" baking dish, and set to the side.
2. In a large bowl, soak dates in rose water for a minimum of 30 minutes. Pour water and dates into a large blender and blend until the dates become pureed and pasty.
3. Pour puree into a large bowl along with hemp butter and stir vigorously to combine the mixture. Gently fold in the remaining ingredients until everything is well combined, and pour into the prepared baking dish. Press down of the mixture to flatten the batter.
4. Place in the fridge to set for a minimum of 2 hours. Cut into 16 bars when ready to serve. Store remainder in an airtight container.

Snickerz Protein Bars

Yield: Ten Bars
Active Time: 10 minutes
Cooking Time: 10 minutes
Chilling Time: 1 hour
Total Time: 1 hour, 20 minutes

Ingredients
Center:
- 9 scoops Brown Rice Protein Powder (Vanilla Flavor)
- ⅔ cup Oat flour
- ½ cup organic coconut peanut butter
- 1 ⅛ cup unsweetened almond milk
- 1 ½ tsp Stevia extract
- ¼ tsp Himalayan Pink salt

Caramel Layer:
- 2 scoops Brown Rice Protein (Vanilla Flavor)
- ½ cup caramel
- 2 tbsp peanut flour
- 1 cup unsalted peanuts, roasted

Chocolate Coating:
- 9 ounces milk chocolate, melted.

Directions
Filling:
1. Line an 8"x8" with parchment paper. Set to the side.
2. In a large bowl, combine peanut butter, almond milk, stevia, and salt. Beat together using an electric mixer using on low speed, and slowly mix in protein powder. Slowly mix in oat flour and protein powder, and mix until well blended.
3. Fold the dough into a ball and dump into the prepared pan and spread and press using a rubber spatula. Place in the fridge to chill for a minimum of 2 to 3 hours.

Caramel Layer:
1. Add caramel sauce to a medium bowl, and stir in the protein powder and peanut flour. Pour over the protein center, and spread the mixture to the outer edges of the protein center, top with peanuts. Place in the fridge to set for a minimum of 30 minutes. Cut into 16 bars and chill for an additional 30 minutes.
2. Remove bars from the fridge, and dip into the melted chocolate. Allow the excess chocolate to drip off. Repeat for remaining protein bars.

Maca Protein Bars

Yield: Ten Bars
Active Time: 10 minutes
Cooking Time: 10 minutes
Chilling Time: 1 hour
Total Time: 1 hour, 20 minutes

Ingredients
- 3 Scoop Pea Protein Powder
- 4 tbsp Maca Root Powder
- ⅓ cup almond butter
- ⅓ cup coconut peanut butter
- 1 ½ cup silvered almonds
- ½ cup pumpkin seeds
- ½ cup ground flax meal
- 2 tbsp chia seeds
- ½ cup sunflower seeds
- ¼ cup organic raw honey
- ¼ cup organic coconut oil
- Himalayan Pink salt, to taste

Cooking Directions
1. Place parchment paper into an 8"x8" baking dish. Set to the side.
2. In a large saucepan, over medium-high heat mix together honey, almond butter, peanut butter, and coconut oil. Mix well until all ingredients are combined. Set to the side and keep warm.
3. Add almonds to a food processor and blend until the almonds reach a coarse chop. Pour into the bowl along with the sunflower seeds, pumpkin seeds, chia seeds, flaxseed, maca powder, and salt. Pour into the saucepan with the almond butter mixture. Mix well to combine.
4. Pour the ingredients into the prepared baking dish, and spread using a rubber spatula. Press down to pack. Place in the fridge and allow to chill for a minimum of 1 ½ hour or until the batter is fully set. Cut into 8 bars when ready to serve.

Nutty Quinoa Protein Bars

Yield: Eight Bars
Active Time: 10 minutes
Cooking Time: 0 minutes
Total Time: 10 minutes

Ingredients
- ⅓ cup quinoa, rinsed
- 16 dates, pitted and chopped
- ⅓ cup walnuts, finely chopped
- ⅓ cup silvered almonds, finely chopped
- ¼ cup dark chocolate (80% cacao)
- ¼ cup coconut peanut butter
- 2 tbsp organic raw honey
- ⅓ cup coconut water
- ⅓ cup rose water

Cooking Directions
1. In a medium saucepan, bring coconut water, rose water, and quinoa to a boil. Reduce heat and simmer for a minimum of 15 minutes. Place in the fridge and allow the mixture to cool for a minimum of 2 hours.
2. Blend dates in a large blender until they begin to form a ball and add to a mixing bowl.
3. Blend almonds, walnuts, dates, and quinoa in a large blender. Pulse until ingredients are well combined. Add peanut butter and pulse again until the ingredients are well combined.
4. With clean hands shape the ingredients into 8 small bars, and place into a shallow plastic container.
5. In a small saucepan, frequently stir together chocolate and honey over low heat until the chocolate is completely melted. Drizzle over the bars and place in the fridge to chill until the chocolate is set.

Chapter 7 – Vegan Protein Bars

The great thing about eating Vegan is that you know you will be eating something that is really good for you. These tasty Vegan recipes are sure to please, and you will be able to fully enjoy the perks of the regular protein bars.

Chocolate Hemp Protein Bars

Yield: Twelve Bars
Active Time: 30 minutes
Cooking Time: 0 minutes
Total Time: 30 minutes

Ingredients
- 5 ounces Hemp Protein Powder
- 1 cup almonds, chopped (divided)
- 1 ½ cup rolled-oats
- ¼ cup cacao nibs, melted
- ⅓ cup black molasses
- 1 tsp cinnamon
- ¼ tsp Himalayan Pink salt
- Unrefined virgin coconut oil

Directions
1. Lightly grease an 8"x8" baking dish with coconut oil.
2. Place ¾ cup almonds and salt in a food processor. Blend until the almonds become a butter or for about 10 minutes. Add oats, molasses, and protein powder. Process the ingredients until a smooth consistency is reached. Press batter into the prepared baking dish. Place in fridge for a minimum of 20 minutes.
3. Pour melted cacao over the protein batter, and cut into 12 bars when ready to serve. Store leftovers in an airtight container.

Peppermint Date Protein Bars

Yield: Twelve Bars
Active Time: 30 minutes
Cooking Time: 0 minutes
Total Time: 30 minutes

Ingredients
- ¼ cup plain Brown Rice Protein Powder
- 1 tbsp raw millet
- 1 cup rolled-oats
- 1 cup packed dates, pitted and chopped
- ¼ cup almonds, chopped
- ½ cup walnuts, chopped
- 2 tbsp cacao powder
- 2 tbsp almond milk
- 2 tbsp large unsweetened coconut flakes
- 1 tsp peppermint extract

Directions
1. Combine all ingredients in a large bowl. And place in a food processor. Dump into a large loaf pan and place in the fridge to set for a minimum of 30 minutes.
2. Cut into 12 bars when ready to serve. Place the leftover bars in an airtight container.

Vegan Red Velvet Protein Bars

Yield: Twelve Bars
Active Time: 30 minutes
Cooking Time: 0 minutes
Total Time: 30 minutes

Ingredients
- 10 scoops Chocolate Pea Protein Powder
- ¾ cup beets, pureed
- ½ cup raw red walnut butter
- ½ cup unsweetened almond milk
- ⅔ cup almond flour
- ¾ cup monk fruit sweetener
- 1 tsp vanilla flavor
- 2 tsp butter flavor
- ⅛ tsp Himalayan Pink salt

Directions
1. Line an 8"x8" baking dish with parchment paper.
2. In a large bowl, mix together beet puree, sweetener, walnut butter, butter extract, and vanilla paste using an electric mixer on low speed.
3. Using a fork whisk together protein powder, salt, and flour. Pour the wet ingredients into the dry ingredients. Mix using an electric mixer until the batter becomes thick.
4. Dump into prepared baking dish and press down to pack. Cover with plastic wrap and chill in the fridge overnight.

Mean Green Vegan Protein Bars

Yield: 12 Bars
Active Time: 10 minutes
Cooking Time: 0 minutes
Total Time: 3 hours, 10 minutes

Ingredients
- 2 tbsp Hemp Protein Powder
- 4 tsp organic Matcha Green Tea powder
- ⅓ cup coconut peanut butter
- ¼ cup silvered almonds, chopped
- 1 cup almond milk
- 1 tbsp rolled oats
- 2 tbsp chia seeds (divided)
- 8 drops lemon flavor
- 1 tbsp lemon juice, freshly squeezed
- 4 tsp monk sweetener
- 1 tsp vanilla extract
- Unrefined virgin coconut oil

Directions
1. Lightly grease an 8"x8" baking dish with coconut oil.
2. Add 1 tablespoon of chia seeds and remaining ingredients into a blender. Blend until the ingredients are fully combined and the batter reaches a smooth consistency.
3. Pour into a medium to large bowl and slowly mix in remaining chia seeds.
4. Set in the fridge to chill for a minimum of 3 hours or until it gels and it reaches a nice pudding consistency. Cut batter into 12 bars when ready to serve. Store remaining bars in an airtight container.

Vegan Gluten-Free Chunky Protein Bars

Yield: 10 Bars
Active Time: 10 minutes
Cooking Time: 0 minutes
Total Time: 3 hours, 10 minutes

Ingredients
- 9 scoops Hydrolyzed Protein Powder (Vanilla)
- 1 cup pretzels, chopped
- 1 ⅛ cup vanilla almond milk
- ¼ cup chocolate chips
- ¼ cup peanut butter chips
- ⅔ cup peanut flour
- ½ cup organic chunky peanut butter
- 2 tbsp monk fruit sweetener
- 2 tsp Stevia extract
- ⅛ cup Himalayan Pink Salt

Directions
1. Line an 8"x8" baking pan with parchment paper, and set to the side.
2. In a large bowl, mix together peanut butter, almond milk, sweetener, stevia, and salt using an electric hand mixer on low speed.
3. In a small bowl, beat together peanut flour and protein powder. Slowly add to the peanut butter mixture while mixing at medium speed. Fold in pretzels, peanut butter chips, and chocolate chips. Pour into prepared baking dish and spread the batter using a rubber spatula. Place in the fridge and chill for 8 minutes or for overnight.
4. Cut into 10 bars when ready to serve, and place remainder in an airtight container.

Seedy Super Strawberry Protein Bars

Yield: 10 Bars
Active Time: 10 minutes
Cooking Time: 0 minutes
Total Time: 3 hours, 10 minutes

Ingredients
- 6 tbsp Soy Protein Powder (Strawberry Flavor)
- ½ cup fresh strawberries, finely chopped
- ⅓ cup chocolate chips
- ¼ cup hemp seeds
- 2 tbsp pumpkin seeds
- 2 tbsp ground flaxseeds
- ¼ cup sesame seeds
- 2 tbsp almond milk
- 2 tbsp organic raw honey
- ½ tsp coconut protein
- 2 tsp ground ginger
- 1 tsp coconut extract
- Himalayan Pink salt, to taste
- 1 tbsp unrefined virgin coconut oil

Directions
1. Line an 8"x8" baking pan with parchment paper.
2. In a medium saucepan, heat coconut oil, honey, and milk. Bring to a boil and immediately remove from the heat. Stir in the chocolate, salt, and coconut extract. Allow to cool for a minimum of 2 minutes.
3. Place pumpkin seeds, chia seeds, flaxseeds, and hemp seeds into a large food processor. Pulse until seeds are finely ground and pour into the chocolate mixture. Stir in protein powder and strawberries. Pour into the prepared baking dish.
4. Place in the fridge and allow the batter to set for a minimum of 2 hours. Cut into 8 bars when ready to serve. Store remainder of the bars in an airtight container.

Conclusion

Protein bars are a convenient way to pump up the protein in your diet. You can enjoy them on the go or as an add-on to your favorite meal. Making a big batch and then storing them for the week in an airtight container is recommended. For an easy, nutritional fix, many people reach for protein bars. The abundant protein content makes it a prime component in an athlete's diet. An essential nutrient-rich protein helps repair and build muscles, which is why many athletes choose protein as an essential part of their diets.

Protein supplementation before, during and/or after resistance-type exercising can increase muscle protein synthesis after a workout and can also inhibit muscle protein breakdown. This doesn't mean that only athletes should be making and eating their own protein bars though! If you want a healthy and hearty snack anytime of day the recipes in this book will surely do the trick!

MY THANKS:

Thank you for taking the time to read this book. I hope you benefitted from it and I hope you will enjoy each and every one of the recipes I have given you. Check out my author central page for more great titles and keep your eyes open for more books from me I the future.

Sincerely,

Ariana Hunter

Made in United States
Troutdale, OR
01/25/2024

17149807R00030